ANTI-INFLAMMATORY DIET FOR BEGINNERS

Simple and Nutritious Meal Plan to Boost Immune System and Heal the Body

Laura R Boyd

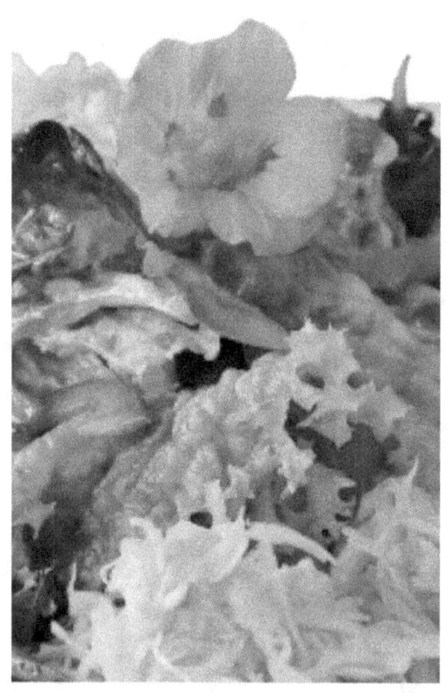

Table of Contents

INTRODUCTION

Understanding Inflammation

Inflammation is a fundamental and sophisticated biological reaction that the human body undertakes to defend itself against damaging stimuli. Far from being a mere annoyance, inflammation plays a key function in the body's innate immune system, acting as a critical mechanism for sustaining health and enabling recovery. However, the key comes in knowing that inflammation, when persistent or unchecked, may shift from a useful activity to a quiet, harmful force within the body.

In its purest form, inflammation is a complicated biological reaction to damaging stimuli such as bacteria, damaged cells, or irritants. This reaction comprises a series of molecular and cellular actions regulated by the immune system. The fundamental objective is to remove the source of cell injury, clear away damaged cells and tissues, and commence tissue restoration.

Inflammation may be divided into two primary types: acute and chronic. *Acute inflammation* is the body's acute and early response to damage or illness. It is a short-lived and localized process, generally resulting in redness, swelling, heat, and discomfort — characteristic hallmarks of inflammation. This sort of inflammation is necessary for the body's defense against infections and injuries and is normally a well-controlled and self-limiting process.

On the other hand, *chronic inflammation* is a protracted and persistent kind of inflammation that can remain for weeks, months, or even years. Unlike acute inflammation, chronic inflammation is frequently low-grade and systemic, requiring a mild and continuous activation of the immune system. This extended inflammatory state is related with a number of ailments, including autoimmune disorders, cardiovascular diseases, and some malignancies.

At the molecular level, inflammation includes a complicated interaction of numerous immune cells, signaling chemicals, and tissue components. White blood cells, particularly macrophages, play an important role in recognizing and removing the cause of inflammation. Chemical mediators, such as cytokines and prostaglandins, organize the communication between cells and govern the inflammatory response.

Chronic inflammation can originate from a variety of factors, including chronic infections, extended exposure to irritants (such as pollution or specific chemicals), autoimmune illnesses, and even excess adipose tissue. Lifestyle factors, such as a poor diet heavy in processed foods, chronic stress, lack of physical activity, and inadequate sleep, can also contribute to the development of chronic inflammation.

While acute inflammation is a natural and important element of the healing process, chronic inflammation poses a substantial danger to health. It is becoming recognized as a contributing factor to various chronic illnesses, including arthritis, diabetes, heart disease, and neurological disorders. Understanding and managing chronic inflammation have become necessary components of preventive healthcare and holistic well-being.

The management of inflammation includes a multimodal strategy that combines medication intervention with lifestyle adjustments. Anti-inflammatory drugs may be given in particular circumstances, but lifestyle variables such as adopting a balanced and nutritious diet, frequent exercise, stress management, and appropriate sleep are key components of a comprehensive anti-inflammatory strategy.

Knowing inflammation is critical to sustaining good health. While acute inflammation is a normal defensive mechanism, persistent inflammation can lead to a cascade of harmful consequences on the body. Recognizing the origins, effects, and treatment techniques for inflammation allows individuals to make educated decisions that enhance overall well-being and longevity.

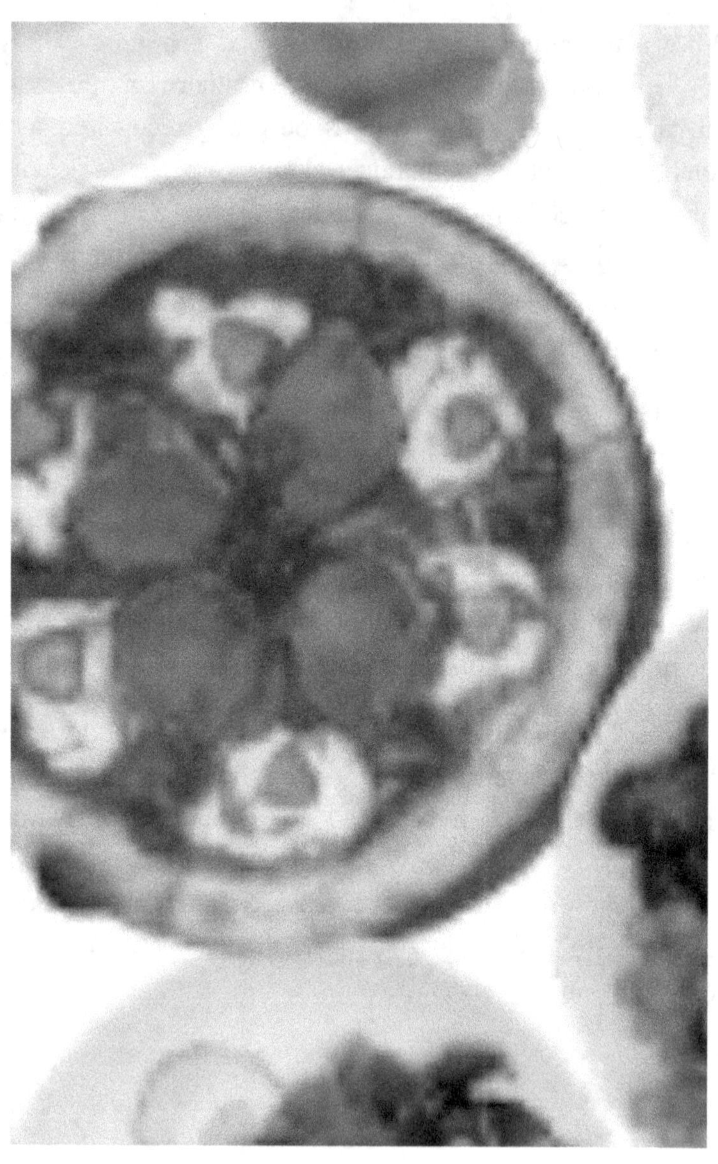

CHAPTER 1

Importance of an Anti-Inflammatory Diet for Beginners

Embarking on the road of adopting an anti-inflammatory diet is not merely a food decision; it's a fundamental investment in one's long-term health and well-being. As beginners go into the domain of mindful eating, knowing the value of an anti-inflammatory diet becomes a guiding principle that goes beyond weight control or transient fads.

Reducing Chronic Inflammation: An anti-inflammatory diet is meant to combat chronic inflammation, a silent contributor to a number of health conditions. By picking foods that actively combat inflammation, beginners may address the fundamental cause of various disorders, including arthritis, cardiovascular diseases, and even some malignancies.

Supporting general Health: Beyond its anti-inflammatory qualities, this diet improves general health by prioritizing full, nutrient-dense foods. Packed with important vitamins, minerals, and antioxidants, these foods give the body the resources it needs to function efficiently, increasing immune function, encouraging organ health, and supporting the body's natural healing processes.

Weight Management and Metabolic Health: For beginners looking to manage their weight, an anti-inflammatory diet offers a sustainable and health-focused strategy. By eating meals that assist to manage blood sugar levels and support a healthy metabolism, individuals can reach and maintain a healthy weight, minimizing the risk of obesity-related inflammation.

Gut Health and the Micro biome: The gut plays a crucial role in immune function, and an anti-inflammatory diet promotes gut health. By combining fiber-rich meals and essential nutrients, beginners may promote a healthy micro biome, providing a harmonious habitat for the billions of microorganisms that inhabit the digestive system.

Energy and Vitality: Adopting an anti-inflammatory diet is not just about what is omitted but also about the lively, nutritious foods that are included. Beginners generally notice higher energy levels and a sense of vigor when they nourish their bodies with complete meals that give prolonged energy and encourage mental clarity.

Long-Term Disease Prevention: Perhaps most significantly, following an anti-inflammatory diet is a proactive step toward preventing chronic illnesses. By managing inflammation early on, beginners can greatly lower their likelihood of acquiring illnesses such as heart disease, diabetes, and neurological problems later in life.

In essence, the relevance of an anti-inflammatory diet for beginners extends far beyond the field of weight control. It is a holistic approach to health that treats the fundamental cause of many health conditions, improves total well-being, and provides a foundation for a bright and disease-free future. As beginners embark on this nutritional path, they unleash the possibility for a healthier, more energized, and resilient existence.

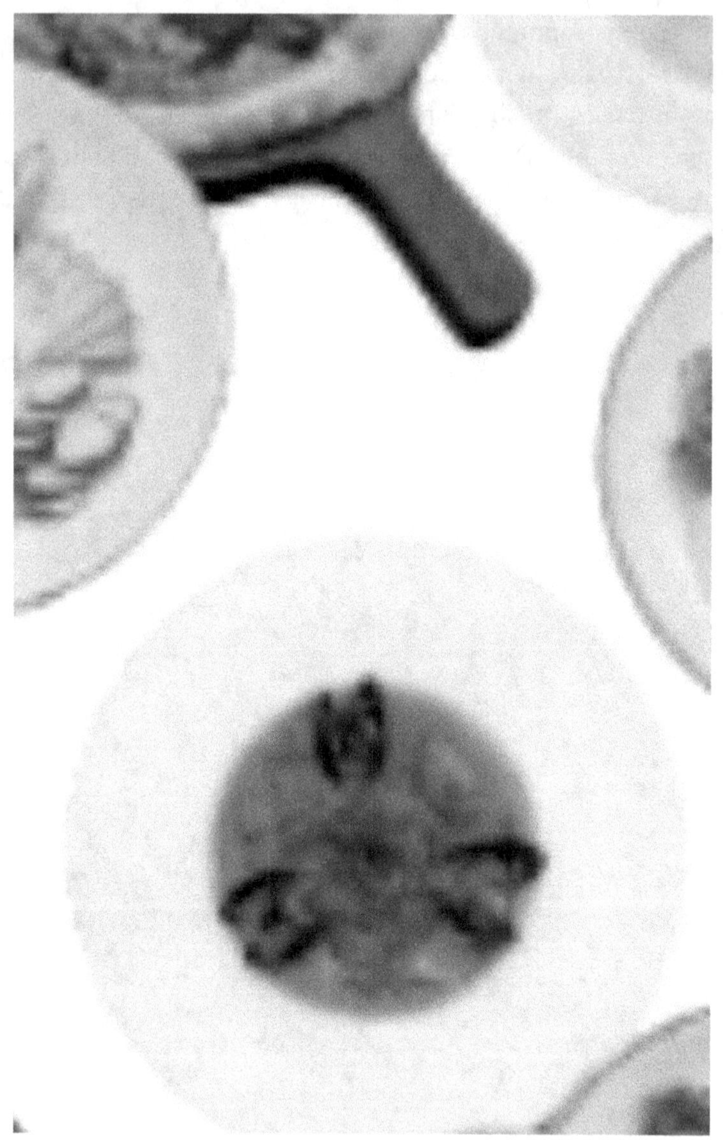

CHAPTER 2

Understanding Micronutrients and Macronutrients

Embarking on an anti-inflammatory food path requires a fundamental grasp of macronutrients and micronutrients, key components that play a critical role in supporting general health and lowering inflammation. For beginners, mastering the principles of these nutrients is important to designing well-balanced and satisfying meals.

Macronutrients, usually known as "macros," are the primary nutrients that supply the energy needed for our body's everyday processes. The three basic macronutrients are carbs, proteins, and lipids. In an anti-inflammatory diet, emphasis is on adding complex carbs like whole grains, which release energy gradually and help regulate blood sugar levels.

Lean proteins from sources such as fish, chicken, and plant-based choices assist tissue regeneration and immunological function. Additionally, healthy fats, found in avocados, almonds, and olive oil, provide anti-inflammatory qualities and assist many biological functions.

On the other hand, micronutrients are vitamins and minerals required in lesser amounts yet are as necessary for good health. These micronutrients play a key role in immunological function, antioxidant protection, and overall well-being. For an anti-inflammatory meal prep, prioritize foods rich in micronutrients like vitamin C, vitamin E, and selenium. These can be found in colored fruits and vegetables, nuts, seeds, and whole grains.

When constructing meals for an anti-inflammatory diet, it's necessary to find a balance between macronutrients and micronutrients. An example dinner would contain quinoa (complex carbs), grilled salmon (lean protein), and a side of mixed berries and spinach (micronutrients). Experiment with herbs and spices like turmeric and ginger, recognized for their anti-inflammatory effects, to boost both flavor and nutritional value.

A good anti-inflammatory diet meal prep for beginners needs a judicious balance of macronutrients and micronutrients. By embracing a range of nutrient-dense foods, individuals may make meals that not only taste wonderful but also actively help to lower inflammation and support general well-being.

CHAPTER 3

How to Meal Plan for an Anti-Inflammatory Diet

Include fruits and vegetables with every meal: Fruits and vegetables are rich in antioxidants and other health-promoting elements that promote immune health and decrease inflammation. Including these antioxidant-rich foods in each meal is a wonderful approach to make sure you get the nutrients your body needs to battle chronic inflammation. Eat an assortment of colors every week, such as dark greens, red and orange fruits and vegetables, beans, and peas each week.

Use healthy fats: Monounsaturated fats found in olive oil, avocados, peanuts, almonds, and seeds aid decrease inflammation. Make these your go-to fats for optimal health.

Add meals high in omega-3 fatty acids: Omega-3 fatty acids are necessary lipids your body needs to create cell membranes. These fats may also help fight inflammation. Fatty fish like salmon, mackerel, and tuna are high in omega-3 fatty acids. You can also acquire omega-3 fats from walnuts, flaxseeds, chia seeds, and hemp seeds, but it is better absorbed in the form that is present in seafood.

Replace refined grains with whole grains: Whole grains like barley, brown rice, and oats are rich in fiber and other nutrients that boost your health and reduce inflammation. Swap out processed grains with whole grains to remain in line with your anti-inflammatory diet plan.

Vary your proteins: Red meat, poultry, fish, eggs, dairy, beans, peas, almonds, and seeds all provide protein. Choose lean sources of animal protein and be sure to incorporate plant sources of protein throughout the week to enhance fiber and vitamin consumption.

Use herbs and spices to add flavor: Herbs and spices are a terrific way to add flavor to cuisine without salt. These taste enhancers also include antioxidants and phytonutrients that may assist your battle against inflammation.

Limit foods rich in saturated fat and added sugar: Foods rich in saturated fat and added sugar cause inflammation. Limiting your intake of these items is suggested when eating to improve better health.

CHAPTER 4

Essential Kitchen Tools and Supplies

Embarking on an anti-inflammatory food journey is a proactive step towards greater health and well-being. To make this shift simple and pleasurable, stocking your kitchen with crucial equipment and supplies is key. Meal planning for an anti-inflammatory diet not only involves thoughtful food selection but also efficient tools to ease the process. Here's a guide to the must-have kitchen essentials for a great start:

Cutting Boards and Quality Knives: Invest in robust, non-toxic cutting boards and high-quality blades for effective chopping and slicing. Opt for separate boards for veggies and proteins to prevent cross-contamination.

Vegetable Spiralizer: A spiralizer is a game-changer for introducing more veggies into your diet. Create noodle-like forms from zucchini, sweet potatoes, or carrots to broaden your dinner options.

Quality Pots and Pans: Stainless steel or non-stick pots and pans are necessary for preparing anti-inflammatory meals without excessive oil. Look for cookware that supports uniform heating and is easy to clean.

Steamer Basket: Steaming is a gentle cooking method that maintains the nutrients in your food. A multipurpose steamer basket allows you to steam a variety of veggies, making dinner prep a snap.

Food Processor: Simplify the process of chopping, pureeing, and mixing with a trustworthy food processor. It's perfect for producing sauces, dips, and homemade dressings without additional preservatives.

Mason Jars and Glass Containers: Portion management is essential to a healthy anti-inflammatory diet. Use mason jars and glass containers to keep preparing goods and meals, increasing freshness and easy visibility.

Herb & Spice Collection: Enhance taste without relying on excessive salt by creating a broad collection of herbs and spices. Include anti-inflammatory alternatives like turmeric, ginger, garlic, and cinnamon for both taste and health benefits.

Measuring Cups and Spoons: Achieve precision in your recipes by using measuring cups and spoons. This assures correct portion amounts and helps you adhere to anti-inflammatory guidelines.

By gathering these basic kitchen tools and materials, you'll be well-equipped to begin on your anti-inflammatory meal prep adventure with confidence and simplicity. The investment in excellent equipment pays off in the form of tasty, healthy meals that boost your entire well-being.

CHAPTER 5

Breakfast Recipes

Turmeric Smoothie Bowl

Ingredients:

1 cup frozen mixed berries

1 banana

1 tsp. turmeric powder

1/2 cup Greek yogurt

1 tbsp. chia seeds

Preparation Method:

Blend all ingredients until smooth.

Top with additional berries and chia seeds.

Nutritional Value:

Approximately 300 calories, rich in antioxidants, fiber, and probiotics.

Cooking Time: 5 minutes.

Quinoa Breakfast Bowl

Ingredients:

1 cup cooked quinoa

1/4 cup almond milk

1/2 cup fresh berries

1 tbsp. honey

1 tbsp. chopped nuts (almonds or walnuts)

Preparation Method:

Mix quinoa with almond milk.

Top with berries, honey, and nuts.

Nutritional Value:

Around 350 calories, high in protein, fiber, and omega-3 fatty acids.

Cooking Time: 10 minutes.

Chia Seed Pudding

Ingredients:

3 tbsp. chia seeds

1 cup almond milk

1/2 tsp. vanilla extract

1/2 cup fresh fruit (blueberries, strawberries)

Preparation Method:

Mix chia seeds, almond milk, and vanilla extract.

Refrigerate overnight, then top with fresh fruit.

Nutritional Value:

Approximately 200 calories, rich in omega-3s, fiber, and antioxidants.

Cooking Time: 5 minutes (plus overnight refrigeration).

Salmon and Avocado Toast

Ingredients:

2 slices whole-grain bread

1/2 avocado, mashed

3 oz. smoked salmon

1 tsp. lemon juice

Preparation Method:

Toast the bread, spread mashed avocado, top with smoked salmon, and drizzle with lemon juice.

Nutritional Value:

Around 300 calories, high in omega-3s, fiber, and vitamins.

Cooking Time: 5 minutes.

Sweet Potato and Spinach Breakfast Hash

Ingredients:

1 sweet potato, diced

1 cup spinach

1/2 onion, diced

1 tbsp. olive oil

2 eggs (optional)

Preparation Method:

Sauté sweet potato and onion in olive oil until tender.

Add spinach and cook until wilted. Top with poached or fried eggs if desired.

Nutritional Value:

Approximately 350 calories, high in antioxidants, vitamins, and fiber.

Cooking Time: 15 minutes.

Blueberry and Almond Overnight Oats

Ingredients:

1/2 cup rolled oats

1/2 cup almond milk

1/4 cup blueberries

1 tbsp. almond butter

Preparation Method:

Mix oats, almond milk, and blueberries. Refrigerate overnight.

Top with almond butter before serving.

Nutritional Value:

Around 250 calories, rich in fiber, antioxidants, and healthy fats.

Cooking Time: 5 minutes (plus overnight refrigeration).

Green Vegetable Omelet

Ingredients:

2 eggs

1/2 cup chopped kale or spinach

1/4 cup diced bell peppers

1/4 cup cherry tomatoes, halved

1 tsp. olive oil

Preparation Method:

Whisk eggs and pour into a heated pan with olive oil.

Add vegetables and cook until eggs are set.

Nutritional Value:

Approximately 200 calories, high in protein, vitamins, and antioxidants.

Cooking Time: 10 minutes.

Coconut and Berry Parfait

Ingredients:

1/2 cup coconut yogurt

1/4 cup granola

1/2 cup mixed berries (strawberries, blueberries)

1 tbsp. shredded coconut

Preparation Method:

Layer coconut yogurt, granola, and berries in a glass.

Top with shredded coconut.

Nutritional Value:

Around 300 calories, rich in antioxidants, fiber, and healthy fats.

Cooking Time: 5 minutes.

Cauliflower Breakfast Hash Browns

Ingredients:

1 cup grated cauliflower

1 egg

1/4 cup almond flour

1/2 tsp. garlic powder

Preparation Method:

Mix grated cauliflower, egg, almond flour, and garlic powder.

Form into patties and cook until golden brown.

Nutritional Value:

Approximately 150 calories, low in carbs, and rich in fiber.

Cooking Time: 15 minutes.

Ginger Infused Green Tea

Ingredients:

1 green tea bag

1 cup hot water

1 tsp. grated ginger

1 tsp. honey (optional)

Preparation Method:

Steep the green tea bag in hot water.

Add grated ginger and honey if desired.

Nutritional Value:

Minimal calories, high in antioxidants and anti-inflammatory properties.

Cooking Time: 5 minutes.

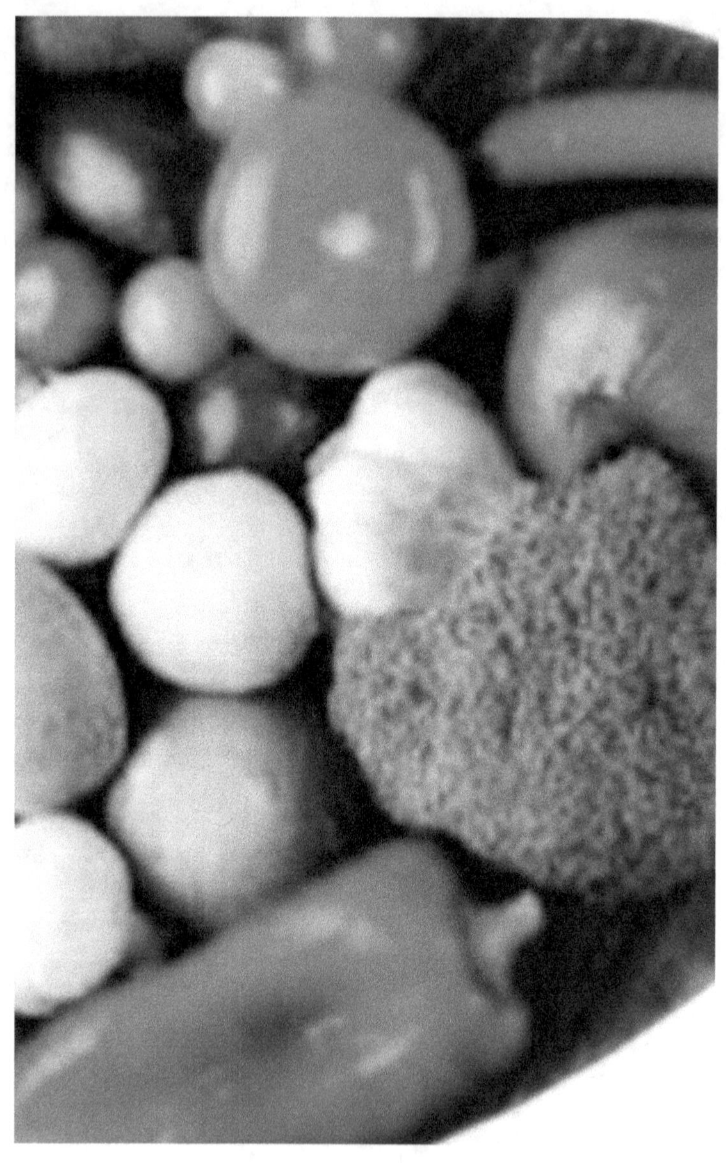

CHAPTER 6

Lunch Recipes

Salmon and Quinoa Salad

Ingredients:

4 oz. grilled salmon

1 cup cooked quinoa

Mixed greens

Cherry tomatoes, sliced

Cucumber, sliced

Olive oil and lemon dressing

Preparation Method:

Combine all ingredients in a bowl and toss with the dressing.

Nutritional Value:

Approximately 400 calories, rich in omega-3s, protein, and antioxidants.

Cooking Time: 20 minutes.

Vegetarian Chickpea Stir-Fry

Ingredients:

1 can chickpeas, drained

Mixed vegetables (bell peppers, broccoli, carrots)

1 tbsp. olive oil

1 tsp. turmeric

1 tsp. cumin

Preparation Method:

Sauté chickpeas and vegetables in olive oil with spices until tender.

Nutritional Value:

Around 350 calories, high in fiber, plant-based protein, and anti-inflammatory spices.

Cooking Time: 15 minutes.

Mediterranean Quinoa Bowl

Ingredients:

1 cup cooked quinoa

Cherry tomatoes, halved

Cucumber, diced

Kalamata olives, sliced

Feta cheese

Olive oil and balsamic vinegar dressing

Preparation Method:

Combine all ingredients in a bowl and drizzle with dressing.

Nutritional Value:

Approximately 380 calories, rich in antioxidants, fiber, and healthy fats.

Cooking Time: 15 minutes.

Tofu and Vegetable Stir-Fry

Ingredients:

1 cup tofu, cubed

Mixed vegetables (broccoli, bell peppers, snap peas)

1 tbsp. soy sauce

1 tbsp. sesame oil

Preparation Method:

Stir-fry tofu and vegetables in sesame oil and soy sauce until cooked.

Nutritional Value:

Around 300 calories, high in plant-based protein, fiber, and anti-inflammatory compounds.

Cooking Time: 20 minutes.

Kale and Walnut Salad

Ingredients:

Kale, chopped

1/4 cup walnuts, chopped

1/4 cup dried cranberries

Olive oil and lemon dressing

Preparation Method:

Massage kale with dressing, then toss with walnuts and cranberries.

Nutritional Value:

Approximately 250 calories, rich in vitamins, antioxidants, and omega-3s.

Cooking Time: 10 minutes.

Lentil and Vegetable Soup

Ingredients:

1 cup lentils, rinsed

Mixed vegetables (carrots, celery, onion)

4 cups vegetable broth

1 tsp. turmeric

Preparation Method:

Simmer lentils and vegetables in broth with turmeric until tender.

Nutritional Value:

Around 300 calories, high in fiber, plant-based protein, and anti-inflammatory spices.

Cooking Time: 30 minutes.

Grilled Chicken and Quinoa Bowl

Ingredients:

4 oz. grilled chicken breast

1 cup cooked quinoa

Roasted vegetables (zucchini, cherry tomatoes)

Lemon-tahini dressing

Preparation Method:

Assemble grilled chicken, quinoa, and roasted vegetables. Drizzle with dressing.

Nutritional Value:

Approximately 400 calories, high in protein, fiber, and antioxidants.

Cooking Time: 25 minutes.

Sweet Potato and Black Bean Salad

Ingredients:

Roasted sweet potatoes, diced

1 can black beans, drained

Red onion, diced

Avocado, sliced

Cilantro

Preparation Method:

Combine sweet potatoes, black beans, red onion, and cilantro. Top with avocado.

Nutritional Value:

Around 350 calories, rich in fiber, vitamins, and anti-inflammatory compounds.

Cooking Time: 30 minutes.

Cauliflower Rice Stir-Fry

Ingredients:

1 cup cauliflower rice

Mixed vegetables (bell peppers, broccoli, carrots)

2 tbsp. coconut aminos

1 tbsp. sesame oil

Preparation Method:

Stir-fry cauliflower rice and vegetables in sesame oil and coconut aminos until cooked.

Nutritional Value:

Approximately 250 calories, low in carbs, and rich in fiber and anti-inflammatory compounds.

Cooking Time: 15 minutes.

Shrimp and Avocado Salad

Ingredients:

Grilled shrimp

Mixed greens

Cherry tomatoes, halved

Avocado, sliced

Cilantro

Olive oil and lime dressing

Preparation Method:

Toss grilled shrimp, mixed greens, tomatoes, and avocado. Drizzle with dressing.

Nutritional Value:

Around 350 calories, high in protein, healthy fats, and antioxidants.

Cooking Time: 15 minutes.

CHAPTER 7

Dinner Recipes

Baked Salmon with Lemon and Herbs

Ingredients:

6 oz. salmon fillet

1 tbsp. olive oil

Lemon slices

Fresh herbs (such as dill or parsley)

Preparation Method:

Preheat the oven to 375°F (190°C).

Rub salmon with olive oil, season with herbs, and top with lemon slices.

Bake for 15-20 minutes until the salmon flakes easily.

Nutritional Value:

Approximately 350 calories, high in omega-3s, protein, and antioxidants.

Cooking Time: 20 minutes.

Vegetarian Lentil Curry

Ingredients:

1 cup lentils, cooked

1 can diced tomatoes

1 onion, chopped

2 cloves garlic, minced

1 tbsp. curry powder

Preparation Method:

Sauté onion and garlic, add tomatoes and lentils, then stir in curry powder.

Simmer for 20 minutes.

Nutritional Value:

Around 300 calories, high in fiber, plant-based protein, and anti-inflammatory spices.

Cooking Time: 30 minutes.

Grilled Chicken and Vegetable Skewers

Ingredients:

8 oz. chicken breast, cubed

Bell peppers, cherry tomatoes, red onion

Olive oil and lemon marinade

Preparation Method:

Marinate chicken in olive oil and lemon, then thread onto skewers with vegetables.

Grill for 15-20 minutes, turning occasionally.

Nutritional Value:

Approximately 400 calories, high in protein, vitamins, and antioxidants.

Cooking Time: 25 minutes.

Quinoa-Stuffed Bell Peppers

Ingredients:

4 bell peppers, halved

1 cup cooked quinoa

Black beans, corn, diced tomatoes

1 tsp. cumin

Preparation Method:

Mix quinoa, beans, corn, tomatoes, and cumin. Stuff into pepper halves.

Bake at 375°F (190°C) for 25-30 minutes.

Nutritional Value:

Around 350 calories, high in fiber, plant-based protein, and anti-inflammatory spices.

Cooking Time: 35 minutes.

Baked Turmeric Chicken Thighs

Ingredients:

4 bone-in, skin-on chicken thighs

1 tsp. turmeric

1 tsp. garlic powder

1 tbsp. olive oil

Preparation Method:

Rub chicken with turmeric, garlic powder, and olive oil.

Bake at 400°F (200°C) for 30-35 minutes.

Nutritional Value:

Approximately 400 calories, high in protein, anti-inflammatory spices, and healthy fats.

Cooking Time: 35 minutes.

Vegetable and Chickpea Stir-Fry

Ingredients:

1 can chickpeas, drained

Mixed vegetables (broccoli, bell peppers, snap peas)

1 tbsp. olive oil

1 tsp. ginger, minced

Preparation Method:

Sauté chickpeas and vegetables in olive oil with ginger until tender.

Nutritional Value:

Around 350 calories, high in fiber, plant-based protein, and anti-inflammatory compounds.

Cooking Time: 20 minutes.

Sweet Potato and Kale Quiche

Ingredients:

1 sweet potato, grated

2 cups kale, chopped

4 eggs

1 cup almond milk

Preparation Method:

Line a pie dish with grated sweet potato. Add kale.

Whisk eggs and almond milk, pour over kale. Bake for 30 minutes at 375°F (190°C).

Nutritional Value:

Approximately 350 calories, high in vitamins, fiber, and protein.

Cooking Time: 35 minutes.

Cauliflower and Broccoli Soup

Ingredients:

1 head cauliflower, chopped

2 cups broccoli florets

1 onion, chopped

4 cups vegetable broth

Preparation Method:

Sauté onion, add cauliflower, broccoli, and broth. Simmer until vegetables are tender.

Blend until smooth.

Nutritional Value:

Around 200 calories, high in fiber, vitamins, and anti-inflammatory compounds.

Cooking Time: 30 minutes.

Spinach and Mushroom Quinoa Risotto

Ingredients:

1 cup quinoa, cooked

2 cups spinach

1 cup mushrooms, sliced

1/4 cup Parmesan cheese

Preparation Method:

Sauté mushrooms, add spinach, then stir in cooked quinoa and Parmesan.

Nutritional Value:

Approximately 300 calories, high in protein, fiber, and anti-inflammatory compounds.

Cooking Time: 25 minutes.

Turkey and Vegetable Lettuce Wraps

Ingredients:

1 lb. ground turkey

Lettuce leaves

Mixed vegetables (carrots, bell peppers, water chestnuts)

2 tbsp. soy sauce

Preparation Method:

Brown turkey, add vegetables and soy sauce, then spoon into lettuce leaves.

Nutritional Value:

Around 350 calories, high in protein, fiber, and anti-inflammatory compounds.

Cooking Time: 20 minutes.

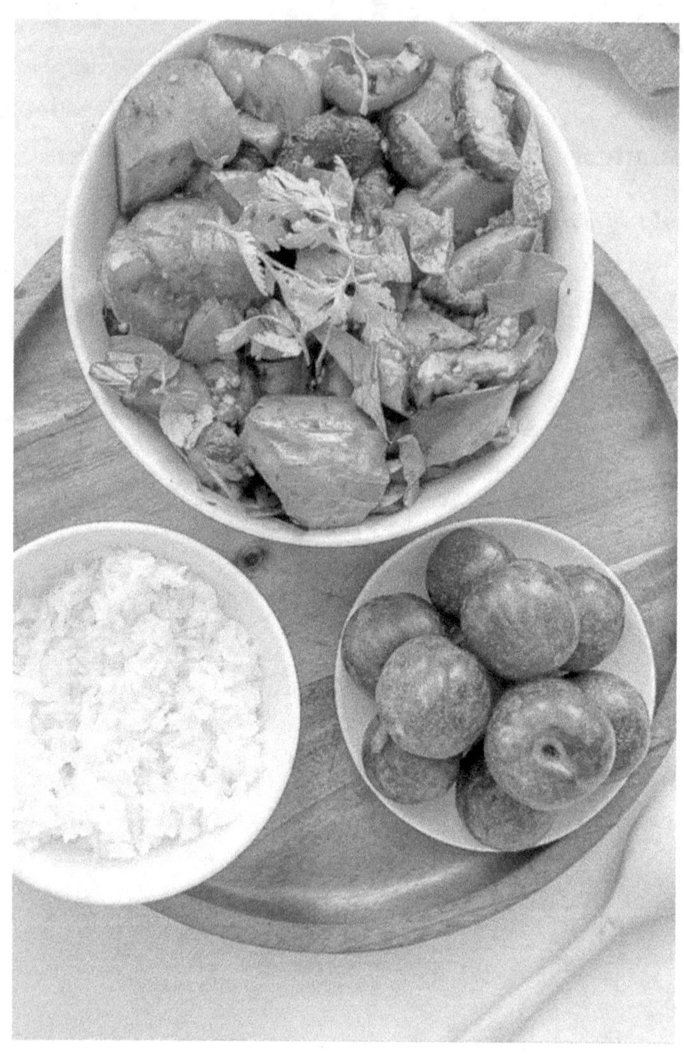

CHAPTER 8

Snacks Recipes

Turmeric Hummus with Veggie Sticks

Ingredients:

1 can chickpeas, drained

2 tbsp. tahini

1 tbsp. olive oil

1 tsp. turmeric

Carrot and cucumber sticks

Preparation Method:

Blend chickpeas, tahini, olive oil, and turmeric until smooth. Serve with veggie sticks.

Nutritional Value:

Approximately 150 calories, high in fiber, protein, and anti-inflammatory spices.

Prep Time: 10 minutes.

Chia Seed Pudding with Berries

Ingredients:

3 tbsp. chia seeds

1 cup almond milk

1/2 tsp. vanilla extract

Mixed berries

Preparation Method:

Mix chia seeds, almond milk, and vanilla. Refrigerate until it thickens, then top with berries.

Nutritional Value:

Around 200 calories, rich in omega-3s, fiber, and antioxidants.

Prep Time: 5 minutes (plus overnight refrigeration).

Almond and Turmeric Energy Bites

Ingredients:

1 cup almonds

1/2 cup dates, pitted

1 tsp. turmeric

1/4 cup shredded coconut

Preparation Method:

Blend almonds, dates, and turmeric. Roll into small balls and coat with shredded coconut.

Nutritional Value:

Approximately 120 calories per serving, high in healthy fats, fiber, and anti-inflammatory compounds.

Prep Time: 15 minutes.

Greek Yogurt Parfait

Ingredients:

1 cup Greek yogurt

1/2 cup granola

Mixed berries

1 tbsp. honey

Preparation Method:

Layer Greek yogurt, granola, and berries in a glass. Drizzle with honey.

Nutritional Value:

Around 250 calories, high in protein, probiotics, and antioxidants.

Prep Time: 5 minutes.

Roasted Chickpeas with Turmeric

Ingredients:

1 can chickpeas, drained

1 tbsp. olive oil

1 tsp. turmeric

Sea salt to taste

Preparation Method:

Toss chickpeas with olive oil, turmeric, and sea salt. Roast at 400°F (200°C) for 20-25 minutes.

Nutritional Value:

Approximately 150 calories, high in fiber, protein, and anti-inflammatory spices.

Prep Time: 30 minutes.

Avocado and Tomato Salsa

Ingredients:

1 avocado, diced

1 cup cherry tomatoes, diced

Red onion, finely chopped

Fresh cilantro, chopped

Preparation Method:

Mix diced avocado, tomatoes, onion, and cilantro. Season with salt and pepper.

Nutritional Value:

Around 180 calories, rich in healthy fats, vitamins, and antioxidants.

Prep Time: 10 minutes.

Spicy Kale Chips

Ingredients:

1 bunch kale, torn into pieces

1 tbsp. olive oil

1 tsp. paprika

Pinch of cayenne pepper

Preparation Method:

Toss kale with olive oil, paprika, and cayenne. Bake at 350°F (175°C) for 10-15 minutes.

Nutritional Value:

Approximately 100 calories, high in fiber, vitamins, and anti-inflammatory compounds.

Prep Time: 15 minutes.

Coconut and Almond Bliss Balls

Ingredients:

1 cup shredded coconut

1/2 cup almond butter

1/4 cup honey

1/4 cup chopped almonds

Preparation Method:

Mix shredded coconut, almond butter, honey, and chopped almonds. Form into balls.

Nutritional Value:

Around 120 calories per serving, high in healthy fats, fiber, and antioxidants.

Prep Time: 20 minutes.

Cucumber and Hummus Bites

Ingredients:

Cucumber slices

Hummus

Cherry tomatoes, halved

Preparation Method:

Spread hummus on cucumber slices and top with cherry tomato halves.

Nutritional Value:

Approximately 100 calories, high in fiber, vitamins, and anti-inflammatory compounds.

Prep Time: 10 minutes.

Mixed Berry Smoothie

Ingredients:

1 cup mixed berries (blueberries, strawberries, raspberries)

1/2 banana

1 cup almond milk

1 tbsp. chia seeds

Preparation Method:

Blend berries, banana, almond milk, and chia seeds until smooth.

Nutritional Value:

Around 150 calories, rich in antioxidants, fiber, and omega-3s.

Prep Time: 5 minutes.

CHAPTER 9

Smoothie Recipes

Turmeric Mango Smoothie

Ingredients:

1 cup frozen mango chunks

1/2 teaspoon turmeric

1/2 teaspoon ginger

1 cup coconut water

1 tablespoon chia seeds

Preparation Method:

Blend all ingredients until smooth.

Nutritional Value:

Around 250 calories, high in vitamin C, antioxidants, and anti-inflammatory properties.

Cooking Time: 5 minutes.

Berry and Spinach Green Smoothie

Ingredients:

1 cup mixed berries (strawberries, blueberries, raspberries)

Handful of spinach

1/2 banana

1 cup almond milk

1 tablespoon flaxseeds

Preparation Method:

Blend all ingredients until smooth.

Nutritional Value:

Approximately 200 calories, rich in antioxidants, fiber, and omega-3s.

Cooking Time: 5 minutes.

Pineapple and Ginger Detox Smoothie

Ingredients:

1 cup fresh pineapple chunks

1/2 inch fresh ginger, peeled

1/2 cucumber, peeled

1 cup coconut water

Ice cubes (optional)

Preparation Method:

Blend all ingredients until smooth.

Nutritional Value:

Around 150 calories, high in vitamin C, antioxidants, and anti-inflammatory compounds.

Cooking Time: 5 minutes.

Green Tea and Blueberry Smoothie

Ingredients:

1 cup brewed green tea, cooled

1/2 cup blueberries

1/2 banana

1 tablespoon honey

1 tablespoon chia seeds

Preparation Method:

Blend all ingredients until smooth.

Nutritional Value:

Approximately 180 calories, high in antioxidants, fiber, and anti-inflammatory properties.

Cooking Time: 5 minutes.

Avocado and Kale Super food Smoothie

Ingredients:

1/2 avocado

Handful of kale

1/2 cup pineapple chunks

1 cup coconut water

1 tablespoon hemp seeds

Preparation Method:

Blend all ingredients until smooth.

Nutritional Value:

Around 250 calories, high in vitamins, healthy fats, and anti-inflammatory compounds.

Cooking Time: 5 minutes.

Cherry Almond Smoothie

Ingredients:

1 cup frozen cherries

1/2 cup almond milk

1/2 banana

1 tablespoon almond butter

1 tablespoon flaxseeds

Preparation Method:

Blend all ingredients until smooth.

Nutritional Value:

Approximately 230 calories, high in antioxidants, protein, and omega-3s.

Cooking Time: 5 minutes.

Mango Turmeric Protein Smoothie:

Ingredients:

1 cup frozen mango chunks

1/2 teaspoon turmeric

1/2 teaspoon cinnamon

1 scoop plant-based protein powder

1 cup almond milk

Preparation Method:

Blend all ingredients until smooth.

Nutritional Value:

Around 300 calories, high in protein, vitamin C, and anti-inflammatory properties.

Cooking Time: 5 minutes.

Cucumber Mint Cooler Smoothie

Ingredients:

1/2 cucumber, peeled

Handful of mint leaves

1/2 cup pineapple chunks

1 cup coconut water

Ice cubes (optional)

Preparation Method:

Blend all ingredients until smooth.

Nutritional Value:

Approximately 100 calories, hydrating, and rich in antioxidants.

Cooking Time: 5 minutes.

Strawberry Basil Bliss Smoothie

Ingredients:

1 cup fresh strawberries

Handful of basil leaves

1/2 banana

1 cup almond milk

1 tablespoon chia seeds

Preparation Method:

Blend all ingredients until smooth.

Nutritional Value:

Around 150 calories, high in vitamin C, antioxidants, and anti-inflammatory compounds.

Cooking Time: 5 minutes.

Blueberry Coconut Chia Smoothie Bowl

Ingredients:

1/2 cup blueberries

1/2 banana

1/2 cup coconut milk

2 tablespoons chia seeds

Toppings: shredded coconut, sliced almonds, and more blueberries

Preparation Method:

Blend blueberries, banana, coconut milk, and chia seeds until smooth. Pour into a bowl and add toppings.

Nutritional Value:

Approximately 300 calories, high in antioxidants, fiber, and healthy fats.

Cooking Time: 5 minutes.

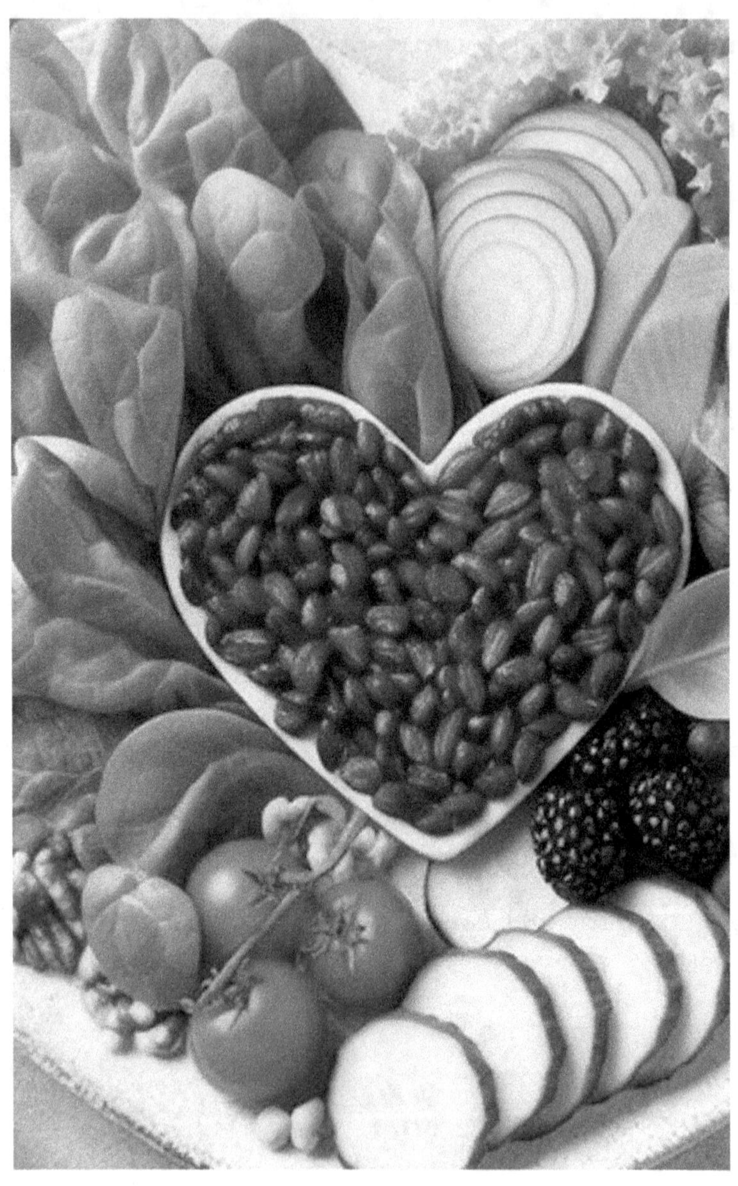

CHAPTER 10

Conclusion

In conclusion, adopting an anti-inflammatory diet may be a transforming journey towards greater health and well-being, especially for beginners trying to make beneficial adjustments in their eating patterns. Throughout this meal plan, we have examined a range of dishes for breakfast, lunch, snacks, dinner, and smoothies, each carefully chosen to integrate components renowned for their anti-inflammatory effects.

The necessity of eating nutrient-dense foods such as berries, fatty fish, leafy greens, nuts, seeds, and spices like turmeric and ginger cannot be emphasized. These components are rich in antioxidants, omega-3 fatty acids, and phytonutrients, all of which play a significant role in lowering inflammation inside the body. By eating whole, unprocessed foods, individuals may harness the power of nature to enhance their immune system, improve heart health, and even ease symptoms linked with inflammatory illnesses.

Moreover, the meal plan stresses a balance of macronutrients and micronutrients, guaranteeing an appropriate intake of key elements including vitamins, minerals, and fiber. This not only contributes to overall well-being but also aids in maintaining a healthy weight and supporting digestive health.

As a tip, it is vital for beginners to approach this nutritional transition cautiously. Start by adding one or two anti-inflammatory meals a day and progressively include more over time. Experiment with tastes, textures, and varied cooking methods to make meals enjoyable and sustainable. Additionally, maintaining well-hydrated and engaging in regular physical exercise enhances the advantages of an anti-inflammatory diet.

Before commencing on any substantial dietary changes, it is essential to speak with a healthcare expert or a trained dietician. They can give individualized counsel based on individual health issues, dietary choices, and particular goals. Monitoring how the body responds to these changes is important, allowing for modifications as needed to enhance the advantages of an anti-inflammatory diet.

In accepting this comprehensive approach to eating, beginners can embark on a journey toward greater health, increased vitality, and a reduced chance of chronic illnesses. The road towards an anti-inflammatory lifestyle is not just about what is on the plate but also about creating a sustainable, pleasant, and satisfying connection with food.

www.ingramcontent.com/pod-product-compliance
Lightning Source LLC
Chambersburg PA
CBHW071058260726
48661CB00006B/2333